WHAT'S NEXT?

NAVIGATING YOUR CHILD'S EXTENDED HOSPITAL JOURNEY

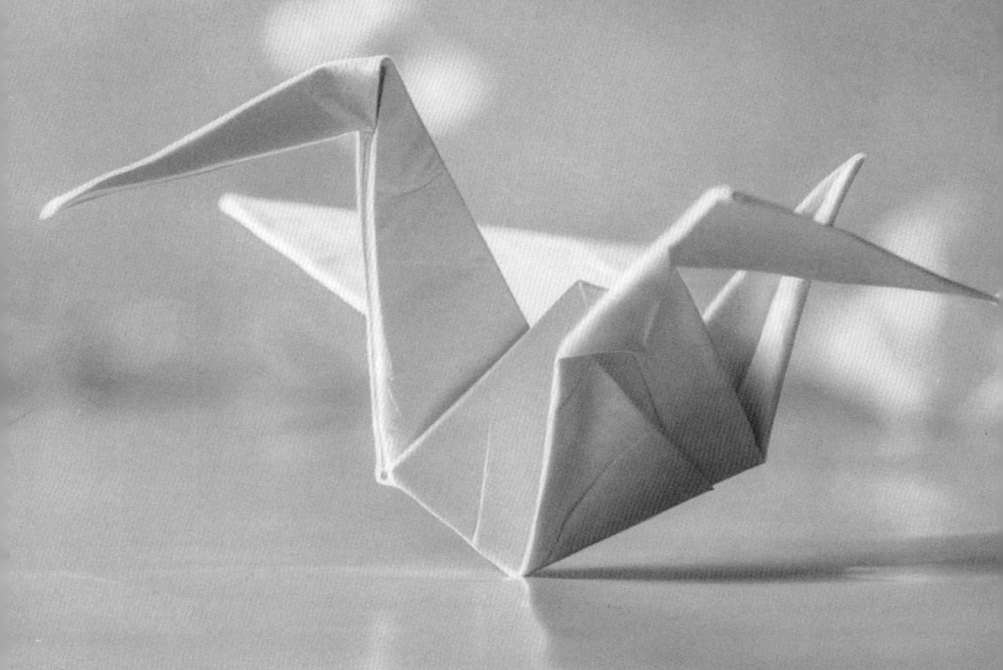

LISA BAKER

Copyright ©2024 Lisa Baker

All rights reserved. No part of this publication may be reproduced in any form, or by any means, electronic or mechanical, including photocopying, recording, or any information browsing, storage, or retrieval system, without permission in writing from the publisher who can be contacted at info@bluehatpublishing.com.

First Print Edition, 2024

Printed in China

Publishing Services: Jodi Cowles, Brandon Janous, and Rachael Mitchell (Blue Hat Publishing)

Cover Design: Tim Marshall (Blue Hat Publishing)

Interior Layout: Jodi Cowles (Blue Hat Publishing)

ISBN (print): 978-1-962674-38-6

ISBN (ebook): 978-1-962674-39-3

While the author has made every effort to provide accurate information at the time of publication, neither the publisher nor the author assumes any responsibility for errors or changes that occur after publication.

Where notated, Scripture quotations are taken from THE HOLY BIBLE, NEW INTERNATIONAL VERSION®, NIV® Copyright © 1973, 1978, 1984, 2011 by Biblica, Inc.® Used by permission. All rights reserved worldwide.

BLUE HAT
PUBLISHING
BOISE • KNOXVILLE • NASHVILLE • SEATTLE
WWW.BLUEHATPUBLISHING.COM

Contents

Dedication	1
Introduction	2
Part I – Navigating the Journey	4
1. The Diagnosis	5
2. Home Away from Home	12
3. Communication with Healthcare Providers	20
4. Communication with Family and Friends	28
5. Caring for Siblings	34
6. Asking for Help	45
7. Advice from Parents	54
Part II - Resources	61
8. The Healthcare Team	62
9. Emotions and Coping	67
10. Child Development	79
11. Final Thoughts	88
References	89
Notes	91

This book is dedicated to my family—you are the joy of my life, and I am thankful for every moment.

To the families

This book would not have been possible without so many families being willing to share their stories. Thank you for your openness and time. What you have gone through has meaning and value, especially to those who are just beginning the journey. And to all the families who are reading this book while sitting in the hospital room or waiting room: Know that you are not alone.

To Juliah

Juliah, I picked you to help with this research not only because of your knowledge but also because of your journey. Nothing is wasted. You are a fabulous social worker—continue to serve with your heart.

Introduction

The word "cancer" can strike fear into any heart, but especially when it relates to your own child. In 2016, our family began a journey that led to our daughter being diagnosed with a Grade 3 Anaplastic Astrocytoma: in layman's terms, a big, scary brain cancer. What followed were multiple surgeries and weeks of hospital stays, plus countless outpatient appointments and therapies in our local children's hospital. We should have been prepared for this. I was a former medical social worker, and my husband was a phyian. But I didn't know how to best help my child during this time. I searched and searched for advice online but was left with nothing practical. I knew that the care team was taking care of her medical needs, but I needed to know how to be a parent. What could I do to make the long stays and uncertainty more manageable for her, how could I also take care of our other daughter, and how could I manage the huge influx of people wanting to help and wanting information? It seemed overwhelming.

We did the best we could and learned some interesting tips and tricks along the way. After our experience, I felt a deep longing to help other parents who were in the same situation. Surely, I couldn't be the only one with these questions? And so began the basis for this book and the research study that has grounded these chapters. Over the past year we have surveyed over 150 parents who had a child with an extended hospital stay, asking the same questions that I posed to myself. We asked about managing the hospital environment, handling communication with both care providers and extended family and friends, how to care for siblings, and how to manage help from others. What resulted was an outpouring of advice and tips reflecting the experience of other parents. While reviewing the data and putting this book together, I decided that we also needed additional chapters on handling emotions and a little about child development. Since these were not the specific questions asked in the survey, these chapters reflect current research as well as some anecdotal content.

The information in this book is directly from our own experiences, the experiences of other parents, and what we know from the research. There was a lot that we learned and a lot we didn't get right, but we got through. I have added a "swing and a miss" section to highlight one of those misses. The thoughts are merely suggestions for you to take or leave, considering what might work best for your family. They come from families in a wide variety of medical settings, from local rural hospitals to freestanding pediatric medical centers. As such, your setting may differ in what you are able to apply. I have started each chapter with an introduction based on our experience. As I am coming from a Christian perspective, you will see references to my faith. My faith was a support to me and remains an integral part of my journey. If you bring a different faith perspective, I am hopeful you will still find value in the experiences of others.

My desire for you as you read through this book is that you will use it as a resource, developed by people who have walked in your shoes, and that it may make the experience a little less overwhelming and give you a little more sense of control as you navigate this journey. If nothing else, I hope it lets you know that you are not alone.

Part I – Navigating the Journey

The Diagnosis

This is the day the Lord has made;
We will rejoice and be glad in it.
—New King James Version,
Psalm 118:24

That verse was never one that I clung to in times of trouble. Yet it was the verse that God put on my heart when I stood in the bathroom of the imaging center at our children's hospital, praying for a verse that would carry me through the day. I welcomed the sterile cold of the bathroom and was grateful that I was alone. I felt shaky and sick to my stomach, immobilized by the words that my husband had spoken to me only minutes before: "It's a brain tumor, and it's big." Our daughter had been having "spells" that had been difficult to diagnose over the past year. They started very minor at first, but by the time we were sent for the MRI they had progressed. She was scheduled to stay overnight in the hospital for a sleep study, but first she was having an MRI that was expected to "show nothing." Instead, it revealed a large brain tumor. It was the first Monday of the school break for the Christmas holiday. She was 17 years old, fully *immersed in her junior year of high school. Instead of going home the next morning, she was scheduled for her first brain surgery.*

I can tell you everything about that night. The feel of the chairs, the smell of the waiting room, the strength of the hugs. I remember a sea of people coming to the hospital, I remember making endless phone calls, I remember her friends coming and playing games and ordering pizza. I remember feeling like I couldn't be physically close enough to either of my daughters. I remember feeling afraid and numb, and I remember an overwhelming sense of God's presence. Time was standing still, and I was very aware in those moments, no matter how scared I was, I was, first and foremost, a mom.

The experience of having a hospitalized child is one that is hard to fully understand unless you have been there. When we surveyed parents, we did not look for families dealing with a certain diagnosis; instead, we were looking for those whose child had experienced an extended hospital stay. Many families experienced multiple stays, dealing with a variety of diagnoses. Some families had complicated surgeries, some were dealing with cardiac (heart) issues, some were dealing with Autism or developmental disorders, some with complicated diabetes, and others cancer. The ages of children ranged from infants to teenagers. No matter the diagnosis, when your family is facing such news, it can be difficult to handle. The fear is real.

The Physical Response

Depending on the age of the child, you may be receiving the news solely on their behalf, or you may be receiving it alongside them. You may feel blindsided, numb, or overwhelmed. It is difficult to know how you are going to get through the next day, or even the next moment. It is common to feel intense sadness or even disbelief, feeling that the news that you just heard could not be correct. A physical response is also common. This could include anger, pounding in your chest or heart palpitations, shaking or trembling. You may notice that you are having trouble concentrating, that you have lost your appetite or begin to have trouble sleeping. Please know that all these feelings are normal and expected. You are trying to deal with something that is very stressful, and the body can react in many ways. The irony is that this time of acute stress is often a time when you must make many decisions: the first of many times you may think that life is not fair. Your mind may already be clouded with a multitude of questions. Why is it your child? Why did this have to happen? What did we miss? It doesn't seem fair.

In our situation we received most news along with our daughter. As a teenager, she was able to receive and process the information, and we tried to be respectful of her developmental stage. We made the choice to let her make as many decisions as possible about her care, and to keep her informed along the way. This was our decision, and each family is different. If I could provide one piece of advice throughout this process it is that *you know your child the best!* At the time of diagnosis, you are entering a world that includes a multitude of decisions, information that may or may not always be understood, a lot of uncertainty, and a lot of new people! It is normal to feel overwhelmed, unsure, and even afraid.

One parent described, *"I felt like I was outside my own body, like I was looking in on someone else's life."* You are not going crazy! You have just been thrown into a world of the unknown. The roller coaster car has left the station, and you are holding on for dear life.

There is no right or wrong way to deal with a difficult diagnosis, which also means that there is no instruction book. What we know about receiving difficult news is that there is a limit to what the brain can process at a time of high stress. That is why it is important to take notes, ask questions, bring others along to hear the information, record meetings with the medical team when possible, and in general, give yourself grace that you may not be able to take it all in. Your medical team can provide a lot of support in this area, so don't be afraid to use them.

Sharing the News

As you are trying to make sense of the diagnosis, one of the questions that comes to mind is "How do I share this information with others," particularly in the early stages? Chapter 3 provides more information on this topic, but the answer is, it depends!

Our daughter was in high school at the time, so we had many "networks" of friends and family and the news travelled fast! You will need to decide who you want to share the information with, and how much detail you want to provide, especially at the beginning when there may be so much unknown. Again, there is no right or wrong in this area! You know your friends and extended family best, and only you can decide how much information you want to share. Remember that it is also okay to take some time by yourself before you share the news of the diagnosis with others. Some people tend to be more introverted and need time alone to process information. If this speaks to you it may be meaningful for you to try to find some time in a quiet area at the hospital to spend a few minutes by yourself, keeping in mind that this is not always possible. Others are more extroverted and like to process with other people. Extroverts may need to keep close to family or friends and talk frequently about what is happening.

Whatever way you choose to share news, being the gatekeeper can be overwhelming. Regardless of your style, recognize that different people process information differently, and it is not unusual to replay the story multiple times as a way of making sense of what you have been told. There is no right or wrong, and it is necessary to give space for those differences, especially when your style may not look the same.

Which brings me to another point, and one that I cannot stress enough: *It is okay to set boundaries*! You are allowed to set limits on who receives information, who can visit, who gets the daily and weekly updates. You don't always need to answer the call, respond to the text, or post an update on social media. You can say no, and sometimes it is necessary to say no. This journey is difficult, and you know what your limits are and the limits of your child and family. Control what you can control and recognize what you can't.

Searching for Answers

Finally, after receiving the diagnosis, it is tempting to go to the internet for answers. I cannot caution enough to be careful about what you find. You may discover helpful information, but you can also get lost down the rabbit hole of reading about other people's experiences that may or may not apply to your situation. There is no question that the internet can be a great resource; however, the content may not always be up to date. The field of medicine is constantly changing and evolving, and new advances are being made. Even "recent" content may reflect research that is several years old. I would encourage you, before you take on the web, to consult with a member of your healthcare team to learn which websites they feel have the best information and are the most helpful. And remember, statistics are numbers that reflect a lot of different scenarios. Your child is an individual, and their journey is unique. Keeping track of their progress will be your biggest guide.

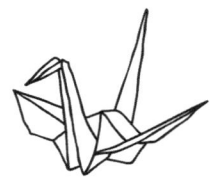

The Diagnosis Highlights

- Hearing the diagnosis may be difficult and bring about a physical response.
- It's okay to set boundaries and take time to process the information.
- Be careful when researching the diagnosis on the internet.
- Know that you aren't alone in this journey.

Home Away from Home

We did the best we could to make her room more home-like. We brought in pictures, flowers, inspirational verses, and lots of special blankets and bedding. People wanted to know what to do, and at times it was difficult to know what to tell them. One day one of her teachers from school asked if she could bring a gift from the classroom. She brought in a large pole that must have had 60–70 colorful origami cranes hanging on fishing line. Our daughter had a large window in her hospital room, and we hung the cranes in the window. During the day the cranes were so beautiful and cheerful. It was special to think that they were made by students in her classroom. At night the cranes were shadows against the lights of the city, flying in the draft of the air conditioner. I don't know what they meant to her, but to me they symbolized life, freedom, and hope for better days. Those cranes still hang in a hallway in our house, validating those feelings. When I see them today, I think of how far we have come.

The hospital environment can be scary for children, even with many children's hospitals doing their best to make it more kid-friendly. Extended hospitalizations are especially difficult, as your world is reduced to a single hospital room. As we interviewed parents, one of the questions we asked was "What did you do to make the setting more home-like for your child?" We received many answers about creative ways that families helped to soften the hospital environment. These included bringing special things to the hospital and decorating like home, keeping special routines, and others. Below are some of the ways families made the hospital environment a home away from home.

Decorating

With extended stays, being able to make the environment more home-like can decrease anxiety and provide a sense of control. Some parents described decorating as a way to continue what is important to the child: *"We decorated the room so it looked just like her bedroom at home. I think that really helped the whole situation and eased her stress. I brought her favorite drawing book because she says she wants to be a painter someday."* Others went to special lengths to add to the environment: *"We brought in some of his play toys, placed photographs of his sister, his Dad, and myself beside his bed, used his favorite bedcover and throw pillow. We made sure his curtains matched those of his bedroom at home. We brought him some of his color books and some crafts he picked during our family vacation. Lastly, we got a photograph of his favorite superhero and placed it on the wall."*

Another parent shared, *"He wore his pajamas instead of a hospital gown when possible. We had a special blanket and lovey that he kept in his bed. If we had notes, gifts, or balloons from friends or family we would set them out for him to see. I utilized the cabinets in the room to store clean clothes like we would have them in dressers at home. I also made a dirty clothes pile for washing when necessary. In the bathroom, I made sure that all the toiletries were given a space—not in travel bags/packages—as close as it would be in the bathrooms at home."*

While each family is different, the suggestions below were common from parents who have been able to make the hospital a little more home-like. Each hospital will have its own policies about what is allowed, so be sure to check before, but below is a list of some of the more common suggestions:

- Bringing photographs of family and friends. These can be placed on the bedside tables, hung in a picture string, or even tacked to the walls and cabinets if allowed.

- Bringing favorite toys and books to read.

- Bringing in flowers, balloons, and small plants to brighten the room.

- Bringing in favorite snacks and food.

- Bringing in entertainment (Gameboys, iPad, electronics, crafting supplies, and board games).

- Bringing in the child's own pajamas and bedding (sheets, blankets, pillows) so they will not need to stay in the hospital gowns.

- Bringing laundry soap from home so that the laundry will smell like home.

    - Note: Sometimes this can be helpful, and sometimes the child may develop an aversion to smells associated with the hospital.

- Bringing in cards that friends and family send, and either putting them on the walls or punching a hole in them and keeping them on a big ring.

- Hanging posters, Bible verses, or inspirational sayings.

- Hanging decorations in the windows.

- Decorating for the holidays.

- Playing music in the room.

- Bringing infant toys such as bouncy seats to keep children entertained out of bed. *"He was under the age of one, so our experience was a little different because he was so little and so sick. But I always packed age-appropriate toys, I always kept him in clean clothes and dressed him for daytime/nighttime. I would bring things for him to do outside of the crib bed, like a bouncy seat and, once a little older, a jumpy thing I attached to the bathroom door opening."*

- Bringing extra tables and small shelves to help with storage. *"We brought items from home that she enjoyed doing such as crafting supplies, board games, movies/laptop. We also brought a folding table for her personal use and a trashcan for her personal use."*

- Lots of visits from family and friends.

- Using Facetime and other electronics to help people visit who cannot come to the hospital.

- Bringing or using a noise machine—this can be very helpful to quiet noise from hallways during times of rest.

- Putting a note on the hospital door to limit visitors when your child is napping.

- Decorating the bed like a castle, race car, or camping tent to make it a special place.

Keeping Routines

Each hospital will have its own set of routines and schedules that will differ from setting to setting. Unfortunately, a hospital stay means that family routines and structure can be difficult to continue. Even so, keeping such routines can go a long way toward normalizing the environment and maintaining a sense of control. When we discussed what parents did to make the environment more home-like, parents frequently spoke of how they kept certain routines that were important to them. These included:

- Maintaining a bedtime routine and reading bedtime stories.

- Prayer time/keeping religious rituals.

- Going for walks.

- Watching sports on TV.

- Playing games as a family.

- Going outside when allowed. *"I came visiting with the dog whenever I could. We would go outside so she could play with him—and this was important."*

- Having family dinner. *"When I asked her sister what she was missing the most she said, 'eating together as a family.' So, I asked the nurses if we could borrow the conference room one night. I cooked dinner at home and brought it in on our own plates. We ate together, just the four of us, outside of the hospital room or the cafeteria. It is one of my favorite memories of that time."*

- Talking to relatives and friends on a set schedule.

- Field trips throughout the hospital.

A Swing and a Miss

Weeks into the hospitalization, I knew that we needed a change of scenery. The "witching" hours were the long hours between dinner and going to sleep. These were the hours where our daughter was most likely to be down, sad, or frustrated. We would often take "field trips," where I would take her in the wheelchair to another part of the hospital to get an Icee, or a Starbucks, or just get us out of the hospital room. One evening, we went outside of the hospital where there was a big green space. I tried my hardest to get her to go across the street to the Waffle House for a waffle. I convinced her that this wasn't illegal, and that there were lots of other patients (mostly from the adult hospital dragging along their IV poles) who went rogue. True, the idea seemed a bit edgy for two rule-followers like us, but I was confident that we needed to bust out. She wouldn't bite and was determined that the nurses were looking for her. I told her that it was okay, that she was with a parent, her legal guardian. She wasn't buying it, and we returned to the hospital. What I craved in that moment was spontaneity, taking a chance to break the routine that we were so deeply engrained in. What she craved was the security of being back in the hospital.

While these are all just suggestions, they can be used to jump-start your own ideas about how to make the hospital more home-like. If there is something you would like to do for your child and you aren't sure if it is allowed—just ask! In our experience, the medical team wants to help you do whatever you can to make the experience better for your child. There may be certain routines that are important to your family that can be implemented, or there may be certain items or visitors that could make a difference in helping your child cope.

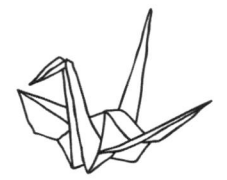

Home Away from Home Highlights

- Don't be afraid to decorate the room to make it more home-like.
- Maintain home routines whenever possible.
- Visitors and family can help pass the time with visits and games.
- If you want to do something and you aren't sure if it's allowed—ask!

Communication with Healthcare Providers

We were fortunate because everyone seemed to know our family, since my husband had worked at the hospital for so long. But even then, a lot of what the healthcare providers told me was hard to comprehend. At times it was because I didn't fully grasp the medical language, but at other times I was so overwhelmed that I couldn't understand. It seemed like the time that they would come to the room would be so short, even though they came in a couple of times a day. I wanted them to stay and tell me over and over until I understood. They were so patient with my questions, but honestly, most of the time, I didn't even know what to ask. The medical updates were very helpful, but what I really wanted to know was just if she was going to be okay, and were we ever going to be back to normal?

Communication with healthcare providers can be one of the more challenging aspects of having a hospitalized child. On any given day, there are many people involved in your child's care, which also means that there are many different people whom you need to communicate with. This list can include doctors, nurses, physical and occupational therapists, child life specialists, social workers, and other counselors, just to name a few. Chapter 8 talks about the many professionals who may be involved in your child's care, and what roles they play on the care team. This mix of providers can be confusing, especially when there are many people who may serve in similar roles. The number of healthcare providers may also vary depending on the type of hospital. For example, a small, rural hospital may have a team that includes just one doctor, whereas a larger, teaching hospital may have a lead doctor as well as other doctors who are training, which may include residents and fellows. All of these are doctors, but each has a slightly different role in your child's care.

In addition, at some hospitals you may find that your doctors rotate, meaning they are only the doctor on that unit for a short amount of time before they switch to another unit. All these factors, coupled with your own feelings of stress and anxiety, can make it very difficult to communicate. One parent shared, *"Making sure that one of us was present at the beginning of the day when rounds were occurring wasn't a challenge, but it was something new we had to make sure we were ready for (taking notes, knowing that this is the time to ask questions or to speak up). It was tricky not knowing sometimes what the right questions were to ask."*

Challenges

When our parents were surveyed, they were asked about the difficulties they encountered when trying to communicate or obtain information about their child's care and diagnosis. Some of these were internal, such as being afraid to ask too many questions, or being anxious about the information they might receive. One parent spoke particularly about the role of being the gatekeeper for information: *"In the first few days we (my husband and I) were together in the hospital, and able to receive the information from doctors and nurses at the same time. At a certain point, my husband had to return to work while I stayed in the hospital. Having to make sure that I was asking all the right questions—insurance questions, repeating all the right information back to my husband later—all the news from the day, and then keeping up with the tremendous amount of new knowledge was overwhelming."* Other parents felt that they didn't have a strong personal connection with the provider, which made it difficult to get information and feel comfortable asking questions.

One of the greatest challenges related to time. Parents felt that sometimes their healthcare provider couldn't give them the time that they needed to ask questions and receive information, because the provider was too busy. This theme was also evident when parents spoke about how it was difficult to always be there at a time when the medical team was available. One parent wrote that *"not seeing the doctor regularly was hard,"* while another parent said that *"there wasn't a stable [regular] doctor in charge,"* meaning that there were many doctors involved in their child's care. However, once the parent-provider collaboration was established, it was very useful: *"Knowing the hierarchy of doctors was helpful. Getting nurses on your side is super helpful, including just being polite. Being organized with med lists and understanding diagnoses is helpful. You make the nurses' job easier being able to communicate about medications. Also, if you have challenges, the nurses will help you by repeatedly paging providers when necessary, paging the attendings (physicians), or explaining different options you might pursue for getting what you need."*

Another significant challenge is comprehension or understanding, not only with language difficulties but also with medical terminology: *"At first everything the doctors were saying to me sounded like the teacher on Charlie Brown was speaking. I had to learn to listen and trust the process of the medical team. That made our situation much easier to deal with."* Some parents also reported that there was a problem in communication due to language barriers, whether it was the parent or provider who spoke a different first language. This problem made it very difficult for parents to understand what was being said about the care of their child. If this is a concern for you, I would encourage you to reach out to see if there is an interpreter in the hospital who can assist. If this is not available, there are several phone services that can provide interpretation. Speak to your healthcare provider or social worker about getting connected with these services.

While the parents surveyed reported several different challenges in communicating with healthcare providers, they also had some very helpful suggestions on ways to improve communication.

Scheduling

Parents said that it was easier to communicate when they knew the schedule of when the providers were likely to be with their child. For example, if the doctors usually stop by in the morning with the rest of the healthcare team, this is a good time to be available—you may hear this referred to as "rounds." One parent reported that being there in person during this time was very helpful in getting to talk with the team.

Emergencies

While we always hope that emergencies won't arise, we also know that realistically, that isn't always the case. Parents shared that they felt more comfortable and appreciated knowing what mechanisms were in place to contact providers in case of emergency. For some this was general contact information; for others it included special call buttons or notifications that were available in the patient room, or centrally located in the hospital. Providing this method of emergency communication was of great help to parents.

Using Friends/Relatives with a Medical Background

Many parents reported that one of their greatest resources for navigating the hospital stay was having friends or relatives who had a medical background. This not only included friends and family who were physicians, but also those with a nursing or other type of therapeutic background. While the friend or relative didn't always know about the specifics of treating the particular diagnosis, just having someone who understood the workings of the medical setting and the different terminology seemed to be very helpful.

Asking Questions

While it can sometimes be tricky, parents overwhelmingly shared that asking questions was one of the most helpful things they could do to communicate with healthcare providers. Throughout this journey, you are going to have many, many questions. Being able to keep track of those questions and ask them of the healthcare provider is essential in moving through the hospitalization. In addition, asking questions allows the provider to know how to best share information, while understanding where you are coming from as a parent. It is extremely helpful to keep a notebook to track questions that you may want to ask as well as to have a place to write down answers to those questions. Some families also referred to using other professionals to provide answers: *"Nurses were super helpful, especially in the very beginning. Once we had some experience under our belt it became easier and more comfortable to ask certain questions to doctors and not feel inappropriate or silly. Once we reached that point, it was helpful to be able to know what was going on, what they wanted to see happen, and what challenges they anticipated for the future."*

Keeping Notes

Just as important as tracking questions is the ability to keep notes. Keeping notes on what was discussed with the care providers is essential. I guarantee that you can forget something that was said as quickly as the provider can walk out of the room! As noted earlier, it can be very difficult for the brain to process information at times, especially in times of crisis. Keeping notes allows you the opportunity to return to those notes to remind yourself about what was said and to also highlight where you need to ask questions. These can also be great ways to track progress with your child and to have concrete responses when you are asked if you have any questions. It can also help to clarify when you may not have heard something correctly or if you need to share information with others, such as family and friends. One parent commented, *"I kept a notebook that I wrote questions in, listed changes in her I noticed, and kept a list of the assistants and nurses as they changed shifts."*

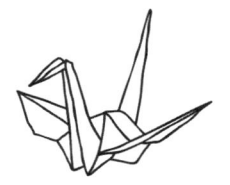

Communication with Healthcare Providers Highlights

- Communicating with healthcare providers and friends and family can be challenging.
- Ask questions and keep a notebook to track answers.
- Be aware of who is involved in your child's care and the role that they play

Communication with Family and Friends

I was not prepared for how much support I needed to give to extended family and friends. On several occasions I had people contact me who felt like they were being left out of the communication loop. These were people who loved and cared for our child, but they felt that there were things about her diagnosis that we weren't telling them. Didn't they know that we didn't know either and we were just as scared? At times it was overwhelming, and at other times I was thankful that I could provide the information, and that I could help ease their minds.

Communication with healthcare providers can be tricky, but so can trying to communicate with extended family and friends. For the most part, the family dynamics that are evident in the normal day-to-day can become exaggerated in times of stress. This can be a good thing or a bad thing. For example, if a family tends to be very supportive and respectful of each other, then they will probably continue that way when dealing with a hospitalization, "circling the wagons" around family members in need. If a family unit is easily stressed, or can become argumentative, this will likely also happen during this time. Know that this is normal. Parents reported that "family drama" was a difficult thing to deal with while they were trying to care for their hospitalized child. One parent noted that the *"constant questioning [from other family members] and the inability to understand questions"* made communication very difficult.

Questions posed by family and friends were often viewed as hard to answer. One parent shared, *"Asking of unnecessary and [seemingly] inappropriate questions really was my biggest challenge."* This was partially because the person answering the question wasn't sure themselves of the correct answer, which led to frustration on both ends. Sometimes medical providers can provide help in answering questions, and parents encouraged reaching out for this type of help. Parents said that it became complicated when family members had different perceptions or viewpoints about how care should be provided, which made the parent second-guess their decisions. Other families reported that they found that they now had a lot of "fake" friends, or friends who were reaching out just to be a part of the attention. One parent noted that *"it seemed like some people were just being nosy while others truly cared."* Distinguishing between these types of people can be tiresome and feel intrusive at times.

When a child is hospitalized, it can also be difficult to attend family gatherings. Parents felt that it was hard to explain why they had to miss family events and felt that no one truly understood why it was important for them to stay at the hospital with their child. One parent commented that some family members insisted on taking the parents out to get a break, but instead of it being a break, it was stressful. The parent shared, *"I know that they were trying to be helpful, and I loved them for that, but it was stressful to sit at breakfast and just think about how much I wanted* to be back with my child, [wondering if they we okay]." From the friend's perspective, that was a way for them to show their love and concern for the whole family, but for the parent it added to the stress.

Finally, many families described a common situation where they were the ones providing comfort to family and friends and managing the fears of others. One parent noted that it was *"difficult to communicate at a time when I was feeling so sad—I just shut down."* We often talk about "emotional or mental bandwidth," which is the ability to hold and process many different pieces of information or mental tasks simultaneously. Finding that extra bandwidth in times of crisis can be exceptionally hard. Shutting down is a common defense mechanism when the brain has reached its limit. It is not uncommon to witness this, especially when one parent is viewed as the caregiver in the larger family unit. The need to communicate with family and friends was described as *"overwhelming and time-consuming."* At these times it can be difficult to shift roles and become the one who needs to be taken care of, rather than the one who provides care to others. One parent shared that they *"wanted to keep things between [them] and [their] family, and . . . kept trying to find a way to tell them without worrying them."*

Time management was also a consideration when sharing information with family and friends. Juggling the hospital schedule with others' work schedules was tricky. Set visiting hours meant that everyone wanted to be visiting at the same time, which was hard when it was a time that the parent felt like they were needed by the child, or if they had limited time to visit.

However, despite these difficulties, parents reported that the support from family and friends was very valuable. Most parents shared that the care they received from family and friends was important and made the families feel like they were less alone. Many reported that family and friends gave very good advice when they could, and that just having family and friends close was helpful. The value of this support was also echoed in answers to other questions as well. Parents appreciated the messages of support that came in many different forms, even when family and friends couldn't be there in person.

Patience

Patience is a virtue! When communicating with family and friends, parents spoke of the need for *patience!* Patience when they were asked the same question many times, patience when they were asked to explain medical procedures, and patience when there was nothing new to report. When parents felt that they had to be the ones providing comfort to friends and family, who were also overwhelmed or not understanding what was happening, it often took patience to respond in a way that was kind. Constantly needing to provide support to others can put a tremendous strain on a family that is dealing with difficult news and a difficult journey, and it can be very helpful to have others who can step in and provide that comfort care.

Overall, parents found many ways to make communication easier. These included the use of social media, group chats, and texts. Some families provided weekly or periodic updates where they were able to decide how much information they wanted to share. Having a point person to provide these updates is extremely beneficial and takes the burden from the family. Video calls using programs such as FaceTime or Zoom were also very helpful in keeping connected and sharing information with family and friends, as well as using sites such as CaringBridge or Facebook for mass updates. Whatever your communication style, realize that there is no right or wrong. You have a right to control the information and the level of communication that feels right for you and your family. There are going to be good days and bad days, and communication may differ depending on the day. It will rarely be perfect, and it's okay to give yourself grace on days when the day isn't going well.

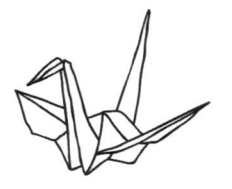

Communication with Family and Friends Highlights

- Social media, group texts, video calls, and online webpages can be useful for sharing information.
- Have patience with yourself and others!
- Recognize that others who love your child may also be looking to stay informed

Caring for Siblings

*T*he day after the "big surgery," the surgeon came in after an MRI and said that he felt the need to go back in to check for another small part of the tumor. We had prepared ourselves for the surgery the day before, but this felt more like an emergency. I felt that we had been blessed that the first two surgeries were without complications, and I was scared that we wouldn't continue to be so lucky. The medical team was prepping the operating room and said they would take her back as soon as it was ready. It all felt too fast. Her younger sister was at school, and I wanted her to be at the hospital with us. I had arranged for a family friend to go to the school to bring her sister to the hospital. I called the school to speak to our younger daughter and she was upset, saying, "I want you to come and get me, please just come and get me." I told her I would, but when I went to tell our other daughter (the patient) who was at the hospital, she said, "Please don't go, I need you here." It was one of the worst moments that I have ever had as a parent, knowing that both of my children needed me to be with them, and not having the ability to be there for both at the same time. It was just as scary for them. My heart was broken in two.

Having a child in the hospital is challenging enough, but also having younger or older siblings at home can add to that challenge. Age, developmental stage, and individual struggles can all be influencing factors in how well siblings can cope with another sibling's hospitalization. The parents we surveyed talked about their feelings on some of those challenges.

Time Management and Juggling Responsibilities

Not having enough time was a very common concern of many of the parents. One parent shared, *"I didn't have enough time to take care of her sibling or family members, because most of my time was spent in the hospital,"* while another shared that *"Having 2 kids is difficult because us parents are always having to choose between kids. [Deciding] who is going to be with which one? That is the hardest thing."*

The difficulty of choosing between children was a very common concern, especially when both were at ages where they needed some level of care. Many families had an older child who was in the hospital as well as a younger child or infant. Multiple children means juggling childcare, infant schedules, and school schedules. One parent wrote, *"At the time of [his] diagnosis, we had a 1st grader and a 3-month-old. Our infant was at every hospital stay, clinic visit, and everything in-between the entire time—that was challenging."* Parents echoed this sentiment, saying that they didn't always have the option to leave a younger child with someone else, which meant that younger child was always in the hospital as well.

Older children, who can be more self-sufficient, may require help with homework, meal prep, and getting to and from school and activities. Several parents commented that their mornings were spent getting their school-age children ready, dropping those children off at school, and then going to the hospital to see their other child. Once at the hospital it was very hard to leave, even when they knew that it was time to pick their other children up from school or daycare.

In addition, this schedule allowed for little time to be able to keep up with things at home. Even simple things like grocery shopping and doing laundry became tasks that were left unattended. As such, juggling responsibilities was demanding, as this parent wrote: *"Inability to multitask was a great challenge, [as] I also experienced a lot of emotional and financial challenges and difficulties"* that made it difficult to get everything done to care for the family.

One family shared that it became so difficult to manage all the responsibilities that they gave temporary custody of their other child to a relative. *"When our son was first born and all his problems started, I had to give my mom temporary custody of my oldest son, so she could take him to school and doctors and sign papers and stuff he needed, so I could stay at the hospital. I took weekends to be with my oldest and mom stayed at the hospital so I could make sure my oldest didn't feel left out and I could make my oldest feel special too. And mom was still there for my oldest son too."* This may seem like an extreme; however, families need to recognize that coping mechanisms may differ from what you are used to doing. Using available resources and being creative can help manage the situation.

Emotional Support

In addition to the concrete needs of siblings, there is also a need to be present emotionally as well. It is sometimes difficult for siblings to understand everything that is happening, because it is also difficult for the adults! A sibling's age and emotional development play a big role in how much information they can receive and process, also differing from child to child. This is another instance of you knowing your child the best, and you will need to make the decisions that you think are correct at the time. I will say that from my years of work as a pediatric social worker, I tend to err on the side of including siblings as much as possible, primarily because when children are not presented with information they tend to make up scenarios in their heads which may be far worse than reality. When a sibling is visiting their brother or sister in the hospital for the first time, it is very helpful to discuss ahead of time what they might be seeing, especially if there is a lot of medical equipment involved. A child life specialist or social worker can also help you navigate these visits and may even be able to meet with the sibling ahead of time to normalize the environment.

Many parents spoke to the need for providing emotional support to the other siblings while balancing the amount or detail of information provided. One parent shared, *"It was very difficult to know what the other sibling needed. I wanted to keep them informed without upsetting or scaring them."* Another wrote, *"The other child was very understanding although they didn't really understand. They were scared because [they saw] me worried."* They further noted that *"the biggest challenge was [the sibling] wondering if Mommy was going to be okay? They didn't really understand, but they never felt like I wasn't there."*

It can also be hard for siblings to see their brother or sister ill, or looking different than they are used to. One parent shared that it was hard for her daughter *"to see her sister being sick and lose her hair,"* while another one shared that the siblings were *"stressed about the state of disease."* As a parent, it can be difficult to know how much to share about the state of the disease, and when to involve other children in difficult conversations. Again, in these situations the best response is often one that is clear and honest, providing age-appropriate information. Child life specialists, social workers, and even chaplains can be a great resource when deciding how much information to share and the best way to handle providing that information and support.

Decreased Attention

When parents need to be with a hospitalized child, it often results in having significantly less time to spend with other children, especially when those children might be experiencing their own difficulties. Not being able to give adequate attention to other siblings can leave parents feeling torn between children who all have different needs. This is especially true with younger children. One parent shared that *"Helping young children understand and be okay with not getting all of the attention they were used to"* was very difficult as a parent. In addition, hospital facilities may not be equipped to accommodate younger children who are visiting. While some children's hospitals do a great job at this, others simply may not have the available space or resources to engage and occupy younger visitors. Or the health status of the hospitalized child may necessitate limitations on visiting and interactions. Having a small bag or backpack with games and toys for the visiting child can provide a special distraction when they need to spend time in waiting rooms or other areas, especially when this "go bag" is only reserved for hospital times.

Routine

Routines are safe and familiar! Try to keep the routine of the sibling intact as much as possible. Children thrive on routine and consistency. At a time when there may be much that is unknown, routines such as school, extracurricular activities, sports, and spending time with friends become very important. Children tend to confide more in their peers than other adults, so allowing time with friends provides an outlet for feelings as well as a support network. This is also a way to provide "protected time" for the sibling. Siblings need an opportunity to continue with practices, games, playdates, and other connections with friends. It is often said that "play is the work of children," and this is very true.

Children of all ages need time to work out their feelings through age-appropriate outlets, and to have times when they are not required to be engaged in hospital activities. For example, a child who has been waiting in a waiting room all day while their sister or brother is having a procedure may be concerned about being late getting to a practice or game later that afternoon. As adults we may think that it is insensitive, when their sibling is having a medical crisis, but take a moment to recognize that the outlet of attending practice is a great way for the sibling to reduce stress, refocus their energy, and have the support of their peer group in a less threatening environment. If you aren't sure what is important to the sibling—just ask them!! Giving a sibling the opportunity to talk about what is important, and not judging the answer, provides reassurance and security, especially when they feel safe in expressing their concerns. If you can't get the sibling to some of these activities, or go watch their game, this is a great job for friends and family who want to help.

Siblings Get Sick Too

At some point, there may be a sibling who gets sick too. Talk about complicating things! It can be easy to dismiss the common cold or minor injury when dealing with a child who is hospitalized for something more severe, but I guarantee that the sibling is also going to be looking for validation. Take this as an opportunity to show the sibling that they are also important. I know, your emotional batteries are already low, but showing attention at this time to a younger (or older) sibling can assure them that they are also loved and cared for. Extra care, attention, check-ins, snuggles, and hugs provide physical and emotional support that offers validation to the sibling that they are an important part of the family, and that they matter. Beware when people say that the other child doesn't have it as bad. Because while that may be true in a medical sense, I have always been of the mindset that suffering is not a competition, and all forms can benefit from some extra care and attention.

Hopping on the Drama Train

Just as you, as the parent, need to manage an influx of people wanting to share in the communication loop or the happenings at the hospital, your child may be experiencing the same thing at school. Especially when the sibling is older, such as middle or high school age. It is not uncommon for a new group of "friends" to pop up and want to be included in the attention. If you sense this is happening, I encourage you to be the gatekeeper whenever possible. Give your child permission to set boundaries and limit the number of people they share information with if it becomes bothersome.

Tell Me About It

Want to know what the sibling is thinking? Ask them! Siblings (of all ages) are curious and typically eager to find out more information. They need an opportunity to process what is happening in the family, even if they don't take advantage of it. Below are some prompts that might get the conversation going:

- How are you doing? Followed up by my favorite question: How are you *really* doing? A great way to get past the automatic "I'm fine" response.

- Tell me what you understand about why your sister/brother is in the hospital.

- What is the scariest part of visiting in the hospital?

- What is the scariest part of having your brother/sister in the hospital?

- If I had a magic wand and could make one thing different, what would it be?

- When you are scared or sad, what makes you feel better?

- If Mom/Dad can't be with you, who is the next best person who makes you feel comfortable? Why?

- Are there things that we used to do as a family that you miss?

- High/low (this a great question for school-aged children): What were the high part of your day and the low part of your day?

- Are your friends doing anything that is really helpful?

- What one question do you wish people would stop asking?

- What do you wish your friends would know about what is happening?

Patience

Patience—here it is again! Patience is important when dealing with siblings, especially when it is hard for them to understand the situation. One parent wrote, *"Our oldest struggled with jealousy for the attention, gifts, and opportunities that were given to her brother following his diagnosis. Trying to teach a young child to not be jealous but to be thankful was very challenging."* This can be true no matter the ages of the children involved, and honestly, sometimes difficult for *all* involved. A parent who had infants in the neonatal intensive care unit wrote, *"My oldest son also needed me, and at his age he couldn't really understand most of what was happening. He knew the babies were in the hospital, but he was never allowed to see them due to cold/flu season (and new COVID protocols). They were almost like unicorns to him during that time."*

So, what is helpful when you lose patience, or feel like you just don't have any more personal resources to handle what is in front of you? Eliminating the situation is not an option, so you need to go to Plan B, which may mean removing yourself for just a moment. I like to call this a "personal" time out! Take a walk, go get a cup of tea or coffee, practice some deep breathing, or just take a moment to gather your thoughts before you respond or react. One day at a time may become one moment at a time, and that's okay!

Being Okay with Getting It Wrong

Which brings me to my final piece of advice for helping siblings: Rely on friends and family to help whenever possible, but know that at some point you are going to get it wrong. Please understand, my dear parents, that I say this with the greatest amount of empathy, because I have been in your shoes. You may not be able to be there when your other child is sick with a cold. You will probably miss something important at school or miss an infant's milestone. You may go home from the hospital after your other children are already in bed, or you may not be able to leave the hospital at all. You are going to feel torn, guilty, and possibly like the worst parent ever (any tears yet?). Know that you aren't! You must give yourself grace in those moments. You are dealing with an unusual situation, and it is probably taking all your resources just to get through the day. That is *okay*—you are showing up! Your other children will be okay, and they may even learn some valuable lessons along the way. Are they things we want them to have to learn? Probably not, but don't forget to look at the growth that can come from difficult experiences. You are one person, and you aren't going to be able to be all things to all people. It will be difficult, you will feel at times like you aren't doing a good job at anything, but I am here to tell you that you are. No one is prepared for this, and we all do the best we can in the moment under extreme circumstances. Grace, grace, grace is what I want to share with you. You will get through—and know that I am sending you a hug.

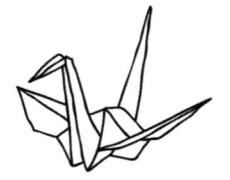

Caring for Siblings Highlights

- Time management and multitasking can be difficult.
- Ask for help from family and friends.
- The emotional needs of siblings will differ depending on age.
- Grace, grace, grace.

Asking for Help

When our daughter had her first "big" surgery she was a junior in high school, surrounded by her "squad" of wonderful friends. During a crisis or time of need we often look towards the adults to provide help and support, but never underestimate the power of your child's friend group. They kept asking how they could help, and finally I had a way. It was December, and with Christmas right around the corner there was still lots that I needed to do at home, even though my greatest priority was to be in the hospital. Christmas was an important holiday in our house, and I was determined to make it as filled with our typical traditions as possible. So, I gave the friends the job of wrapping gifts! I put the gifts for each family member in large bags, loaded the friends up with paper and ribbon, swore them to secrecy, and set them loose in our house while I was at the hospital. They did a beautiful job of tackling this time-consuming task. When they were finished, I couldn't thank them enough. It was then that one of them came up to me and confessed that there was a very good chance that they had mixed up the bags, and they weren't exactly sure that the correct names were on the packages. Those girls will never fully appreciate how meaningful and helpful that simple task of wrapping was to me, and how it made Christmas morning even more special knowing that there was a surprise in every package! I still smile when I think of this memory.

When one of your children is in the hospital for an extended time, it is natural for family and friends to want to help as much as they can. Up until this point I was the one who always was extending help, and I loved doing it. I often felt that it was one of the gifts I had been given—to serve others. However, now I was (and had to be) on the receiving end of the help. For me it was a very humbling experience, and one that didn't come easily. I have always been a "do it on my own" person, so this was not natural. We had so many friends and family who wanted to help, but at times it was difficult to know what we needed. I had to let my guard down and let them help. The help was very tangible, needed, and welcomed. I also knew that it was what they needed to do to show their love and support.

Emotional Support

When we surveyed parents, there were different ways that people received help. While some ways included concrete acts such as food and financial support, there were also many who felt that the emotional support was just as important. Parents shared that *"Encouraging words, prayers, and emotional support was really helpful,"* and even advice, as one parent wrote: *"Financial support, encouragement, and the different words of advice really helped a lot."* Emotional support came in many different forms, including friends and family giving of their time in many ways. Visits may appear to be a concrete way to show support, but the recognition that visits meant that people were giving of their time was extremely appreciated. Parents noted, *"Everyone made time to come with good tidings and good wishes. It was helpful and made a remarkable impact"* as well as *"They devoted their time, finances, and emotional support to my child and the whole family."* All of these were varying forms of emotional support.

Hospital People

I am a "hospital person." My years as a medical social worker have made me very comfortable being around people who are sick and injured, families who are in distress, and people who are in crisis. I have a high tolerance for unpleasant sights and smells, and have no trouble being around medical equipment that is serving in multiple capacities to handle bodily functions. If you have a hospital person in your family or friend group, they are easy to recognize. They will sit all night in an emergency room, keeping you company, bringing you drinks, and making sure that your parking ticket is correctly validated. They will camp out during a 12-hour surgery and speak in hushed tones, asking you every few minutes if you need something to eat. They are a whiz at finding which vending machine has the best coffee and learning the quickest way to score a meal pass to the cafeteria. They are ready with an encouraging word, a kind prayer, or just holding your hand. These are your go-to people when you need support while in the hospital, especially when filling those long hours of surgeries or lengthy procedures.

On the opposite end are your non-hospital people. These people panic at the sound of a siren, become squeamish at even the thought of blood or bodily fluids, and are convinced that every hospital germ is concentrated in the square foot surrounding their space. They may never come visit, and if they do, they are obviously uncomfortable. Do not discount this group! This is your "home team." These are the people who are still there for you emotionally—just at a distance. They are great talkers when you need distracting and great listeners when you need to share. They love concrete tasks such as driving carpool, taking over pet care, and running errands. They are ready and willing and spring to action when you have a need; they are dependable and always follow through. Don't ask non-hospital people to come to the hospital—it is out of their comfort zone. They may do it, but only because they love you, and their blood pressure will be up the whole time. But this is what is important: You will need *both* groups to help you through.

Taking Care of the Day-to-Day

All types of support are needed and appreciated, especially when there are other children or family members at home who need care. One parent wrote, *"Checking up on my child, showing love, as well as the gifts and errands they ran for me [was very helpful]."* And this help can take many different forms. One parent wrote that friends were able to help in multiple significant ways that were important to the family: *"We had a church friend who set up a SignupGenius. The sign-up form included yard work, grocery shopping, laundry duty, home visits, and a meal train. We also had a handful of friends that were able to come over on early morning spinal tap appointments to help our oldest get on the bus—super helpful!"* Another parent appreciated *"Yard work, housekeeping, gift cards, and having friends decorating my house for Christmas one year."* These comments reflect that while the focus of the family is on what is happening in the hospital, there are still day-to-day errands and tasks that need to be accomplished. One parent wrote, *"They assisted me at home to care of the pet and also called to check on me and my child,"* sharing both the emotional and the concrete nature of the help being provided.

Meals

I live in the South, which is home to the understanding that food is the universal love language and that no self-respecting funeral, luncheon, bridal shower, or Easter Sunday is complete without deviled eggs. Alan D. Wolfelt wrote that "Food is symbolic of love when words are inadequate," and I believe this to be true. If I can't help fix it, I will feed you. This sentiment was frequently echoed by parents, whether that was meals provided in the hospital or at home. One mother shared the importance of friends who provided *"Meals to my other children when I couldn't be there or just didn't have the strength to cook because I was busy taking care of my sick child."* And it wasn't just the meals that were appreciated. One parent shared, *"A snack gift basket was the best item we received. Super helpful and we never realized we could use it,"* while another commented that one of the best gifts they received was a large container of fruit: *"We had been eating whatever we could get our hands on, so none of the choices were very healthy. The fruit was a pleasant change that we appreciated."* And eating in the hospital can be expensive! Many parents spoke of the financial burden of needing to eat multiple meals a day at the hospital or in nearby restaurants; in such cases the meals or area gift cards were extremely helpful.

Don't Underestimate the Little Things

The hospital floor that we were on had a kitchenette in the waiting area where families could get drinks, along with a refrigerator and microwave.

In the mornings when he was coming in to work, my husband would often drop off food from home so that I didn't need to eat hospital food. His favorite was to bring me oatmeal that he had made, so that I would have a good breakfast. It may seem like a little thing, but it meant the world to me, not only for the health and energy benefit of eating good food, but also the way that it made it feel very much like we were a team, and the way that the simple act felt very caring and nurturing.

Other Suggestions

Many of these quotes reflected that parents often didn't know what to ask for, or what would even be helpful. It can be difficult when people ask "What can I do?" and you don't know. But recognize that people want to help, or they wouldn't ask. Don't be afraid to be specific. If you want someone to just be present with you, tell them that you would really love to take a walk and grab a cup of coffee. If you are worrying about laundry building up at home, don't be afraid to ask for laundry help. If you are worried that your pets aren't getting enough attention when they are accustomed to daily walks, ask someone to take them to the dog park or go by and walk them daily. In my experience, friends and family know that there is little they can do to help take away the pain and challenges of having a child in the hospital, and they welcome opportunities to help.

Below is a list of common suggestions that we received from parents about what help from friends and family they found to be most useful:

- Signup lists for meal trains, visiting hours, and household help

- Being in charge of group chats and updates

- Carpooling and taking other children to activities

- Playdates for other children
- Helping other children with homework and projects
- Lawn care
- Collecting the mail
- Pet-sitting and pet walking
- Snacks for the hospital
- Help with laundry at home
- Gift cards to nearby restaurants
- Gift cards for meal and grocery delivery services
- Planning time to come and sit with the hospitalized child so parents can run errands or attend sibling events
- Hospital visits from friends and family
- Gas cards and parking credit
- GoFundMe for financial assistance
- Morning coffee break with their favorite coffee
- Cleaning services for the house, especially prior to discharge
- Bringing a care package for the child or parents
    - This can include:
        - Snacks

- Toiletries

- Entertainment items (magazines, coloring books, puzzles)

- Encouraging quotes and messages

- Comfort items such as fuzzy socks, blankets, etc.

- Small notebooks, cards, and pens

- Laundry detergent or special soap

- Basket to help organize items in the hospital room

This list is just suggestions of what other families found to be helpful, but don't hesitate to ask for something that isn't listed. Think about the support that is the most important to you and your family and don't be afraid to ask. If the support you need is a listening ear and for someone to say that they are praying, tell people how important that is to you. If you need tasks at home completed, your non-hospital people will probably jump to the ready! And above all, if you are typically not comfortable asking for help, allow yourself to be vulnerable and open up to others. It also means a lot to the person extending the offer.

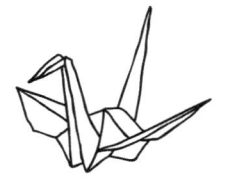

Asking for Help Highlights

- It can be difficult to ask for help.
- Help can include emotional and concrete support.
- Don't be afraid to ask specifically for what you need.
- Friends and family want to help—let them!

Advice from Parents

I have always believed that people do the best they can do at the time. It can be difficult to give advice, because each person's journey is different. For me, I can easily say that I wish our daughter, and our family, never had to experience this medical emergency, or the challenges that came after. But at the same time, I truly believe it made us stronger as a family, more caring, and more empathetic to others experiencing a similar situation. My faith was tested and strengthened in ways I didn't know were possible. I have been able to share our story with others, and for me, it was a testament to the importance of faith and the grace of God. Others have different faith perspectives, and I respect all those differences. The one piece of advice I can give is to take one day, and one moment, at a time. Don't project too far into the future, and give yourself a tremendous amount of grace along the way. You are going to do things great, and you are going to get things wrong. All of this is okay. For me, I often look back at that time and think, "That was really hard." But at the time, I was managing just what was in front of me and working to get through the day. You are stronger than you think, and you can handle more than you ever thought you could.

When faced with a difficult situation, we often want someone who has gone before us to give us the "magic solution." What did you learn? What advice do you have for getting through? These are the reflection points, the points where you look back on the experience and think "I wish I would have known. . . ." The parents who were surveyed were open and honest about their advice to others and what they had learned along the way. In order to preserve their responses, I have chosen to just list them, so that you can take what speaks to you.

What do you wish you had known at the time that you didn't know?

- I wish I would have known how exhausting it is to be in a hospital for an extended stay. Allow yourself to have downtime. If volunteers come around, go outside for a walk. If someone offers to bring food, take it. If you can get someone to do laundry for you, accept it.

- I wish I would have known that the hospitalization of a child as a parent is never easy. [There are] a lot of sleepless nights involved.

- I wish I would have known to let [the staff] know that if you need a few moments to yourself, the hospital has people who can watch your child while you get a breather.

- I wish I would have known that taking care of a sick child requires maximum attention and help from family and friends; don't ever reject their help and support.

- I wish I would have known that I needed to stay strong. It's not going to be easy but you have to be strong so your child can stay strong, [they] watch you.

- I wish I would have known that it's OKAY to ask for help. It's OKAY to not be OKAY. These times are stressful, but you are not alone. Take a minute, get the cup of coffee or tea. Step out for a minute to decompress. Because you can't pour from an empty cup.

- I wish I would have known to always make your child comfortable no matter their illness. That one smile goes a long way by healing them at heart.

What advice do you have for other parents?

- Pack snacks! We learned quickly to bring an extra bag for snacks. It's a small thing, but food gets expensive!

- It's OKAY to ask for something. It's OKAY to ask for a second opinion. No one is there to judge, only help.

- Take time to breathe! Take it one day at a time and [don't be afraid] to be present.

- Be confident in the fact that you know your child better than anyone, remember that. Do not let anyone make you feel like you are wrong when it comes to your child or that you are trying too hard. [Be willing to] fight for what they need.

- We had the agreement in the very first few days of [our son's] diagnosis, there was no way we could go forward and look days, months, years ahead—it was too much. We had to focus on going one day at a time. It was the only way to keep worry for the future to a minimum. Tackle one day at a time.

- Be consistent and never stop believing in your family.

- Love always, life is short.

Connection

- I wish I would have known to connect more with my child during the treatment. It was easier to be clinical and just take care of what needed to get done, much harder to be emotionally available for my child.

- Develop relationships with the parents around you. They are going to be your biggest support. Get involved with local organizations like Smile-a-Mile and ATeam. It is a great way for you and your child to have fellowship and support each other.

- Find someone who can guide you through the ins and outs of your stay. And do your research—ask friends, family, Facebook, everyone. Find out what's possible for care.

- Find you a good support group of special needs families who know what you are going through—they will understand and support you the most. Provide information to your family about your child's conditions and let them ask questions. Listen and explain it to them so they will understand what you and your child are going through on a daily basis.

What have you learned?

While no one wants to go through these experiences, there is often a chance that learning occurs during the process. This can be a recognition of qualities that you didn't think you or your family had, or it can be the development of wisdom that takes you to another level. There is so much power and wisdom in the statements below, and I hope that you will recognize yourself in some of these. The last question that parents were asked was "What have you learned?" and they responded:

- I have learned to be patient.
- I learned how to reach out to people.
- I learned how to give care to my child.
- I learned that love heals.
- I learned that I have a lot of courage.
- I learned to be open-minded.
- I learned that life can happen to anyone.
- I learned that the medical practitioners are really working hard to save people.
- I learned that communication matters a lot.
- I learned that [this experience] has widened my knowledge about everything that happened during that period—and it has also given me boldness to talk about it with others.

- I learned the power of relationships.

- I learned that being present counts more than being a perfect parent.

- I learned to make communication a priority between me and my kid and my family members.

- I learned that emotional health is just as important as physical health.

- I learned that if you have a question or a problem, ask multiple people/staff for their advice on a solution. You may not find the right answer until you have asked many people.

- I learned that life can change quickly, but we are stronger than we realize.

- I learned that it's OKAY to ask for help. And it's OKAY to not always be in control of everything, because we can't predict everything.

- I learned that I have become stronger. I understand more what other parents go through, and I have a special place in my heart for special needs kids and their family. It's hard, but it is always worth it no matter what you go through.

- I learned that when you adapt yourself to an environment, you will overcome any obstacles or challenges you may encounter.

- I learned to just be the best version of yourself and be strong for your child.

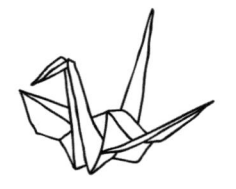

Advice from Parents Highlights

- Ask for help
- Trust your instincts
- Take one day at a time
- Connect with others
- You are stronger than you think!

Part II - Resources

The Healthcare Team

Resident, doctor, attending, therapist? The number of providers that can be involved with your child can be overwhelming! Below is a list of common care providers that you may come across during your stay. For the most part the provider will introduce themselves and the role that they play, but if they don't, don't be afraid to ask.

The Doctors

Not all doctors are created equal! You may have one doctor who is the primary provider, or you may have multiple doctors who are involved in your child's care. These are some of the titles you will most often see:

Attending Physician – A board-certified physician who has completed all their medical and specialty training. They are eligible to work independently and are often the doctor "in charge" or the one supervising the other physicians.

Fellow – A physician who has completed medical school and residency and is receiving further training in a specialty area.

Resident and Intern – Residents and interns have completed medical school and are continuing their training under the supervision of an attending or fellow. The first year after medical school, residents are referred to as interns.

Specialty Areas – Attendings, fellows, and residents may also have training in the following specialty areas, so you may see a general physician as well as a doctor with this specialty training:

Adolescent Medicine – This specialty area provides care to teenagers. They can work with primary care and mental health as well as handle issues of reproductive health.

Allergy and Immunology – This specialty area has special training to diagnose and manage problems such as allergic reactions; diseases of the immune system; stem cell, bone marrow, or organ transplants; and some gastrointestinal disorders that are a result of food and immune reactions.

Cardiology – This specialty area has training in diagnosing and managing disorders that are related to the heart.

Dermatology – This specialty area provides care to patients who have skin disorders. This many include birthmarks, skin infections, skin cancer, and some vascular disorders.

Emergency Medicine – This specialty area provides care in the emergency department to any child or adolescent who comes in. This care can include anything from minor infections to severe trauma.

Gastroenterology – This specialty area has training in diagnosing and managing problems of digestive health. This can include issues with the GI tract, liver, and pancreas, as well as some nutritional disorders.

Hematology-Oncology – This specialty area has training in diagnosing and treating different types of cancer and blood disorders. They may also oversee stem cell transplants.

Infectious Disease – This specialty area diagnoses and cares for patients who have an infectious disease. This can include diseases such as influenza, measles, malaria, and otherwise unexplained infections.

Neonatology – This specialty area cares for premature and full-term infants up until the point that they are discharged from the neonatal intensive care unit. A neonatologist may be present during a high-risk delivery to assess the infant and determine if they need further care.

Nephrology – This specialty area provides care to patients who have problems with the kidneys. This may include chronic (ongoing) kidney issues as well as kidney transplants.

Neurology – This specialty area provides care to patients who have disorders of the brain, spinal cord, and nerves. This can include problems such as cerebral palsy and chronic headache.

Pulmonology – This specialty area has training in managing breathing disorders and disorders of the lungs. This may include asthma, lung disease, lung transplants, and cystic fibrosis.

Rheumatology – This specialty area provides care to patients who have disorders such as arthritis, lupus, and some autoinflammatory diseases.

The Nurses

Just as doctors have different levels of training, nurses also have different levels. These include:

Certified Nursing Assistant (CNA) – This team member does not have a degree in nursing, but has at least a high school diploma and completed a specialty training program. They assist the patient to provide care such as help with bathing and feeding, and other activities.

Licensed Practical Nurse (LPN) – This team member performs tasks such as administering medicines, taking blood pressure, and starting IVs. These care providers have completed a training program that typically lasts at least a year. They are supervised by a registered nurse.

Registered Nurse (RN) – This team member has the primary nursing responsibility for patient care. An RN has completed a bachelor's degree in nursing and may have additional training in a specialty area. They have also passed a rigorous clinical exam.

Advanced Practice Registered Nurse (APRN) – These nurses have completed a master's degree in nursing and have passed a certifying exam. They may specialize as a Nurse Practitioner, Certified Nurse Midwife, Clinical Nurse Specialist, or Certified Registered Nurse Anesthetist.

Other Team Members

In additional to physicians and nurses, there are other providers who may be routinely involved with your child's care.

Social Worker – A social worker in a medical setting typically has at least a master's degree in social work and often has an additional clinical license. They support patients and their families to address social and emotional needs. They may assist with discharge planning, crisis intervention, supportive counseling, bereavement services, education, and identifying resources.

Child Life Specialist – A child life specialist is a provider who helps the patient understand their illness or injury, as well as any procedures that the child may need to have. A child life specialist has at least a bachelor's degree and often a master's degree. They provide developmentally appropriate support and education to the patient, family, and siblings.

Chaplain – Many hospitals have a chaplain who is either available full-time or can come to the hospital if requested. Chaplains provide spiritual care to patients and families regardless of that person's faith perspective.

Psychologist – A psychologist is a member of the healthcare team who provides support, assessment, and mental health counseling to patients and families. They have a doctorate degree and advanced training. A psychologist may use assessments or other tools to help diagnose the patient's level of functioning in the home, hospital, and school and provide services based on those assessments.

Physical Therapist – A physical therapist works alongside the healthcare team to provide rehabilitation to patients after an injury, illness, or other disorder. They work with the movement of the child, helping them to develop balance, coordination, endurance, flexibility, and strength.

Occupational Therapist – An occupational therapist works alongside the healthcare team to provide rehabilitation to help a child with life skills such as dressing themselves, feeding and swallowing, writing and fine motor skills, and school-related tasks.

Speech Therapist – A speech therapist is also called a speech-language pathologist. A speech-language pathologist helps children work on their verbal and non-verbal skills. This may even include working with feeding and swallowing, especially with infants.

Emotions and Coping

*Y*ou think it is going to be over when you leave the hospital. You have survived the experience and you are so happy to just be home. There were many "dark" moments during our hospital stay: the day of the initial diagnosis, the day that she was in so much pain and we couldn't get it to lessen, the urgent trips to MRI to make sure that her brain wasn't swelling or bleeding, the fear of the unknown. But there were also good moments as well: her first smile after surgery, hearing her make a joke, watching her younger sister and her friend ride up the elevator with surgical masks on, because they thought people would think they were nurses (they are both nurses now), watching my daughter take her first steps as she relearned how to walk (I think I may have cried more then than when she took her first steps as a baby). And even now, smiling as I hear her complain that the adult hospital doesn't let you watch videos during an MRI like the children's hospital.

For the most part I think we did okay—not perfect, but okay. But what I didn't recognize was how quickly, even years later, I could get back to those "dark" places. As a person of faith, I have tried my hardest to choose "faith over fear," but it never comes easy, it is always intentional. Every subsequent MRI, every headache, every time I hear the words "I don't feel good," I can go back to those dark places quicker than the blink of an eye. But it is getting easier. Sometimes a headache is just a headache, and there are *times when my head overrides my heart to reinforce that we are not in the same place we were years ago. The more time that passes, the more positive reports and clear MRIs we get, the more it helps to reassure this mama's heart. But the heartache is real, the fear is real, the simple moments of joy are real, and the roller coaster is real—keep hanging on.*

There is a reason that the hospital stay is often referred to as a roller coaster ride. Believe me when I tell you, dear families, that you are going to feel all the feels. Worry, guilt, anger, stress, grief, and yes, even possibly joy at times. And this will all take a toll on you and your child. This is the hard part of the journey, the part that you can't fix with a simple anything, and the part that will be different day to day. It is exhausting. Some days you need to remind yourself to breathe, and some days you might feel like you can't handle one more thing. These emotions are evident in the hospitalized child and siblings as well, so it is important that we recognize what the symptoms are so we can use different tools to help cope.

Stress in Adults

What it looks like:

While some symptoms of stress are easy to recognize, others can be more difficult, and can show up as symptoms of other common problems. This stress can be caused by worry about your child's health, worrying about siblings, changes in relationship with your spouse or significant other, difficult family dynamics, and financial problems due to decreased work or medical bills. Some common signs of stress in adults include:

- Being irritable

- Being impatient

- Difficulty concentrating or making decisions

- Feeling anxious or overwhelmed

- Having a sense of dread

- Feeling depressed

- Having racing thoughts or feeling like you can't turn your brain off

- Headaches

- Muscle aches

- Not sleeping well

- Difficulty breathing

- Panic attacks

- Loss of appetite or increased appetite

- Not wanting to engage with other people

What can help:

When you begin to notice stress symptoms, there are coping skills that may be helpful. These include:

- Eating well
- Going for a walk or exercising if possible
- Calling on your support systems
- Asking someone to sit with your child so you can take a break
- Journaling
- Maintaining religious rituals
- Getting plenty of sleep (difficult if you are not sleeping well)
- Making sure you are communicating well with your significant other
- Deep breathing or meditative exercises
- Speaking to other parents or professionals

What doesn't help:

When we are stressed, it can be tempting to go to things that may seem to help initially but are actually harmful. These include:

- Eating too much
- Eating foods that aren't healthy (high fat or high sugar)

- Drinking excessive amounts of caffeine
- Using drugs or alcohol

Some days are going to be better than others, and you may notice different emotions within the same day. This is completely normal, and your capacity to deal with these changes will differ from day to day. Do what you can and give yourself grace when it is just too much. Hang on and recognize that tomorrow is a new day.

Stress in Children

Children also experience stress. Stress in children can look like stress in adults, but there are some differences.

What it looks like:

- Irritability
- Acting out
- Stomach aches
- Trouble sleeping
- Difficulty concentrating
- Decreased appetite
- Fighting with family and friends
- Being fearful

- Nightmares

- Regression (ex: a child that never wets the bed may start wetting the bed)

- Thumb sucking

- Hyperactivity

- Clinginess

- Crying

- Withdrawal

These signs and symptoms will differ depending on the developmental age of the child. Remember that the child is also feeling the stress, whether they are the hospitalized child or a sibling. Children may also have difficulty verbalizing their emotions, so it can be helpful to ask questions that might help identify the source of the stress. And remember that it is okay to share what you are also feeling to normalize the thoughts of the child. You can say, "Mommy wishes that you were home in your own room too, but let's see what we can do to make this a better place to be while we are here," or "When I feel sad, I find that it is really helpful to talk to some of my friends, so I don't feel alone." Identifying feelings and sharing solutions can empower children to recognize both the stressors and the solutions in themselves.

It is important to keep a lookout for these symptoms, or any behavior that is not typical of your child. Because you are also under a lot of stress, it can be easy to react, but try to take a step back and see what is happening that is causing the stress. Is it worry about a diagnosis or upcoming procedure? Is it frustration at being in the hospital room or having the change in routine? Is it feeling helpless about not being able to change the situation? Trying to determine the cause of the stress can help to identify what might be able to help. And remember that it can be difficult for children to be able to regulate their emotions. If it isn't always easy for adults, it is less so for children.

What can help:

Just like adults, children need outlets to help release their stress. Parents can attempt to provide these in many forms, including:

- Teaching deep or "box" breathing to get through stressful moments

- Allowing visits from family and friends

- Play—this is very important for younger children who may have difficulty expressing emotions

- Journaling

- Visiting hospital activity rooms

- Making time for fun when possible; this can include doing art, listening to music, playing board games, etc.

- Talk, talk, talk it out

- Letting the child make decisions whenever possible

- Modeling healthy coping

- Finding online support groups that are age-specific

- Seeking support—the social worker, child life worker, or psychologist can help

- Guided imagery

- Muscle relaxation

- Changes of scenery

  - Get out of the hospital room if possible—take a walk, visit another part of the hospital, let your young child get their "wiggles" out.

What doesn't help:

- Getting angry at behavior changes

- Allowing the child to escape to social media or video games for an extended period

- Thinking it will go away

Crying

Have you ever heard the expression "You just need a good cry"? That is because there are psychological and physiological benefits to crying. Research shows that crying releases endorphins, which are also called the "feel-good" hormones in the body. Endorphins can relieve physical and emotional pain and can bring about release of negative emotions. Crying can improve mood, help sleep, relieve stress, ease pain, and help regulate emotions. So don't be quick to shut down those tears. A good cry can be just what the doctor ordered.

Hugging

I am a hugger, but many people are not. Either way, just like crying, there are benefits to hugs as a physical way to release emotional tension and stress. Like crying, hugs also release those "feel-good" hormones, which can elevate mood and decrease stress. Hugs can build trust and provide a sense of safety and security. A good hug can lower blood pressure, decrease heart rate, and relieve muscle tension. And don't be afraid to hang on! Studies show that the longer the hug, the greater the benefit. You can hug until you feel the other person relax. This will benefit not only the other person, but you as well.

Grief and Loss

My dear families, if your hospital stay ends with the loss of your child, please know that there are no words I can write that will ease this pain. That journey requires a different book. However, it is important to know that grief can rear its ugly head in many different forms, not only in the physical loss of a child. The signs of grief are very similar to the signs of stress, and can include anger, guilt, anxiety, depression, difficulty making decisions, difficulty sleeping, and much more. But while you may not be experiencing grief in the traditional sense, you are experiencing loss, and it is okay to grieve those losses. You may be grieving the loss of the health of your child, or your dreams for your family as you realize that the future may look different. You and your child may be grieving the loss of your previous lifestyle, your routines, and your independence as now your days are structured by tests, procedures, and therapy appointments. For some of you, the stress of the hospitalization may take a toll on relationships with significant others, and you may be grieving the loss of that support and interaction. You may have family and friends who pull away, and you may be coming to grips with the fact that those groups look different now. All of these are legitimate types of losses, and it's okay to take the time to recognize them as losses and grieve accordingly. This is the same for your child, and it can be especially confusing for them as they have a harder time managing those "big" emotions.

If you find yourself in these areas, please use some of the techniques that have been discussed in this section. Know that these feelings are normal, and there is no right or wrong. Recognizing these emotions as a form of grief is healthy, and allows an opening to process those feelings and move on to a better place.

Life after the Hospital

So, you made it! Your child has been discharged, and you are back home. So why are you still feeling so overwhelmed? Because what you and your child have been through is overwhelming, and sometimes traumatic. It can take some time to process all that has happened, and the stress can linger. You may not be able to go back to your normal routine. Home life may look different, and you may still have a schedule filled with outpatient appointments. The same rules that apply to stress in the hospital apply here.

The research has shown that many children exhibit signs and symptoms of post-traumatic stress disorder after an extended hospitalization. This can show up as increased anxiety, especially around future doctor appointments; increased stress; emotional distress; sleep problems; and behavior problems. These symptoms can be mild to more severe, depending on the child and the hospital experience. You can help your child by helping them talk through their feelings and understand what has happened and what might happen in the future, especially if there are regular, ongoing outpatient appointments, tests, and procedures. Helping a child learn relaxation techniques and other positive outlets can provide coping skills to guide them when these feelings arise.

While this response is normal, I would encourage that, if you find yourself or your child experiencing these symptoms, you consider reaching out for some professional support. The hospital social worker, psychologist, or even child life specialist may be able to provide a referral to a counselor who specializes in this area. Sometimes these symptoms will resolve on their own the further away you are from the hospitalization, but prolonged symptoms may benefit from some additional support. Remember, the transition back to "normal" may take time, and in some cases, you may be thrown back on the roller coaster in the future. Remember to take one step at a time, give yourself grace, and know that you are not alone!

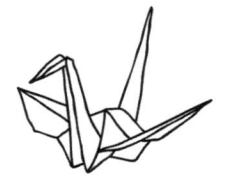

Emotions and Coping Highlights

- The whole family can experience signs of stress.
- Rely on positive coping strategies rather than harmful ones.
- You can still experience stress after coming home.
- Seek professional support if your symptoms continue.

Child Development

I think that every parent wishes that children came with an instruction book that tells us how they are thinking, feeling, and growing along every step of the way. While no two children are ever alike, there are people who have studied the way children grow and learn, and what is important to children at every stage of growth. This section on child development is meant to give just a little insight into the inner workings, and to help parents understand what children are working through from a developmental perspective. It is important to note that these theories are very general guidelines, which can look different from child to child. You might be able to recognize some of these ideas in your own child, or it's also okay if you don't. Children may not always be in these stages at the ages specified, due to delays in cognitive development or delays due to medical conditions.

When it comes to child development, there are many different theories about how children learn and grow at each stage. Each theory has its own ideas, but one I have found particularly useful is the theory of psychosocial development from Erik Erikson. This theory outlines eight stages of development, with the first five stages covering the periods from infancy through adolescence. I have found that these stages are easy to apply to the hospitalized child, and can give some insight as to what might be helpful from a child development perspective.

Stage 1: Trust versus Mistrust (infancy to 18 months)

Oh, the poor baby! They are safe and sound inside their mother, and all of a sudden, they are thrust into the real world, without the warmth and security they felt only moments before. During this time, the primary task of infancy is to develop trust in the world around them. They gain this trust by developing relationships with caregivers, seeking to find reassurance and validation at every step of the way. So, what does this look like? Babies communicate their needs through their cries. When caregivers respond to their cries, infants learn to trust that their needs will be met. Different cries have different meanings, from hunger to need for comfort and affection. This is the earliest form of communication and learning about reciprocal relationships. Infants who do not receive this reinforcement often learn that they cannot trust the world around them. However, imagine the environment of the neonatal intensive care unit. There are many caregivers on the healthcare team, but they are responding to the needs of many infants, and some of those needs are more urgent than others.

Helping children at this stage

Infants who are hospitalized at this stage may not always be able to receive an immediate response to their needs. This can be for medical reasons, or simply because they may be separated from their primary caregiver. One way that you can help your infant is to be present as much as possible. Provide physical comfort and touch, holding or rocking when allowed. Provide comfort during procedures if you are able to do so. Bring things from home such as soft toys or special blankets if allowed. Record yourself reading a story, or provide soft music that you may have listened to before delivery. These are all ways to show the infant that their needs are important, and that they can trust the world around them. Remember, though, that there may be times when it is not possible to provide that level of comfort and care. You may not be able to be present as often as you would like, or you may also be taking care of other siblings at home. Do the best you can at the time, and give yourself grace when you can't.

Stage 2: Autonomy versus Shame and Doubt (toddler to three years old)

"I do MYSELF!" Oh, if I had a nickel for every time my hand was pushed away by one of my girls declaring that, whatever task was at hand, she certainly did not need my help! Children at this stage are yearning for independence and autonomy. They want control over anything and everything. And as exasperating as it can be at times, it is allowing that sense of control that helps children build independence and confidence in their own abilities. Individual identities are forming, and children begin to take charge in small circumstances in order to learn what they can and can't accomplish on their own. Children who aren't given these opportunities to be successful—or navigate failure—can develop a sense of shame and doubt. There needs to be space for trial an error as children learn from their mistakes and grow in self-confidence.

Helping children at this stage

Opportunities to help children at this stage can be limited in the hospital setting, but it can still be accomplished. If your child is able, this is a great time to visit playrooms and allow them to make some decisions on their own. Can they choose what clothes or pajamas to wear? Can they help decorate their room? Can they make decisions about what their favorite snacks are? Allowing children at this stage to exert their own ideas and independence whenever the opportunity presents can help build the foundation for confidence. Provide comfort when they are appearing scared or fearful. Provide outlets for play, and maintain routines whenever possible; setting structure and normal boundaries can establish a sense of security. And provide a lot of encouragement along the way. Be honest, but discuss procedures in simple, age-appropriate language, recognizing that you may need to repeat things multiple times.

Stage 3: Initiative versus Guilt (preschool to three to five years old)

Jean Piaget, a famous child psychologist, once said that play is the work of children. This is never truer than in Erikson's third stage of child development. Children at this stage are often already in preschool or early childhood education programs where they are learning about the world and social interactions through play and other skill-building activities. They are learning about relationships, the complex world of friends, and controlling experiences. They use observation, take instruction, and rely on trial and error to develop skills, building a sense of accomplishment. These children may also begin to exhibit feelings of shame or guilt when they have acknowledged doing something wrong or displeasing others. For example, they may feel guilty for getting sick, and feel like they have done something wrong. Children who feel guilty are often reluctant to try new things for fear that they will not be successful.

Children at this stage may also exhibit signs of "magical thinking," or beliefs that their actions have caused something to happen, when in fact it had nothing to do with them. It is important to look out for this in siblings, as a young sibling who gets annoyed at their brother or sister may think that they caused an illness. Imagination looms large and can be both a comfort and a source of stress.

Helping children at this stage

This is a great stage to take advantage of a child's natural inclination to work things out through play. Playing with your child, and allowing them to play through scenarios that are stressful, can provide insight into what they are thinking or worried about. Talk about emotions that they may be feeling, including anger, sadness, and fear, and reassure the child that they did not do anything to cause the situation. Maintain schedules and routines when possible, and know that this is a great time to use art, coloring, and music as outlets to express emotions and relieve stress.

Stage 4: Industry versus Inferiority (elementary/middle school to eleven years old)

Oh, those lovely middle school years. The years when peer groups are so important, and the development of social and emotional skills takes a front seat. Children in this stage are yearning for parental support as they navigate this new world. Relationships in this stage still center on family in the early years, moving to more peer-centered relationships as the child increases social independence. Children are looking for ways to develop confidence through school, friend groups, and sports. They are gaining new skills and accomplishments. Success leads to feelings of competence and strong self-esteem, while failures can lead to feelings of inferiority, or feeling like they are not good enough.

Helping children at this stage

A child who is hospitalized at this stage may be keenly aware of differences, and may be self-conscious about their illness or different abilities. While children at this age may have a better understanding of their illness, it is still important to provide honest information while encouraging questions. Continue to reassure the child that they did nothing to cause this situation, and help them identify feelings such as anger, sadness, and doubt. Provide the child opportunities to be in control of their environment by seeking input on how to decorate their room or chosen activities when allowed. Help the child use coping techniques such as creative outlets, like art and music, and help them find ways to connect with peer groups when possible. Relaxation exercises and journaling can be additional tools for coping at this stage. This is definitely a "one foot in and one foot out" stage of development. Don't be surprised if your previously very independent child seeks more attention and affection from you to connect and feel safe. Even at this age, they may not always be able to verbalize feelings, seeking other ways to gain reassurance.

Stage 5: Identity versus Confusion (teenagers to 18 years old)

Of all the stages to be parenting a hospitalized child, I would say that the teenage years can be the most challenging. The teenage years are when adolescents truly develop their own sense of identity and being, as well as a sense of self. They begin to solidify their goals and values and shape their social environments around these goals and subsequent peer groups. A prolonged hospitalization can challenge this developmental stage, as it varies from "the norm" of what life should be like. At this stage, school and peer groups are very important, and relationships with others (including family) are key. Adolescents begin to make decisions about their identity, which includes social, emotional, and physical characteristics. They decide how much they want to be alike to and different from those around them, which can sometimes result in identify confusion as they navigate their way. Adolescents are trying to figure out how they fit in the larger world around them and are often highly influenced by peers and societal pressures. Social media is very impactful as teens navigate these challenges and seek a sense of belonging.

Helping children at this stage

Children at this stage are keenly aware of what is going on and the impact on their social and emotional lives. At this stage, it is a delicate balancing act of providing support while respecting privacy. Respect that older teens may want time to talk with healthcare professionals on their own. Encourage your child to talk about their concerns and feelings, but recognize that they may be more comfortable doing this with their peer group. Help the child recognize the range of emotions they may be feeling, and provide positive mechanisms to cope. If possible, arrange for friends to come and visit and help them maintain connections. Help your child identify appropriate resources if they want to get more information, and ask the healthcare professionals if there are any local or virtual teen-based support groups that might be available.

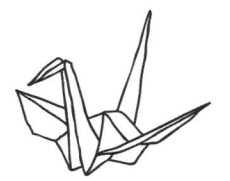

Child Development Highlights

- Your child's needs differ depending on their developmental stage.
- Developmental stages are just guidelines to help understand behavior.
- Your child is unique—do what works best for them!

Final Thoughts

I hope that the words on these pages have left you with a little bit of comfort and maybe some direction to help you navigate these waters. I believe in you and your ability to be the parent that your child needs you to be. You are coming to this armed with everything you know about your child, and the unique relationship that is yours alone. I hope you find strength in yourself and those around you, and that you give yourself an abundance of grace along the way.

From one parent to another,
~ Lisa

References

Children's Medical Center at UMass Memorial Health. (n.d.). *Helping children cope with health care experiences.*

Clemens, J. (2020). Fostering resilience in hospitalized children. *Pediatric Nursing.* 46 (4), 204-206.

Daughtrey, H.R., Lee, J., Boothroyd, D.B., Burnside, G.M., Shaw, R.J., Anand, K.J.S., & Sanders, L.M. (2024). Stress symptoms among children and their parents after ICU hospitalization. Journal of Intensive Care Medicine. 39(4), 328-335. https:/doi/10.1177/08850666231201836.

Delvecchio, E., Salcuni, S., Lis, A., Germani, A., & Di Riso, D. (2019). Hospitalized children: Anxiety, coping strategies, and pretend play. *Frontiers in Public Health*, 7:250. .

Hendy, A., El-sayed, S., Bakry, S., Mohammed, S.M., Mohamed, H., Abdelkawy, A., Hassani, R., Abouelela. A., & Sayed, S. (2024). The stress levels of premature infants' parents and related factors in NICU. *SAGE Open Nursing*, 10, 1-10. .

Ng, N.K.Y., Dudeney, J., & Jaaniste, T. (2024). Parent-child communication incongruence in pediatric healthcare. *Children,* 11 (39).

Rogers, A. (2022). *Human Behavior in the Social Environment: Perspectives on Development and the Life Course*. Routledge: New York.

The National Child Traumatic Stress Network. (n.d.). *At the hospital: Helping my child cope*.

The National Child Traumatic Stress Network. (n.d.). *At the hospital: Helping my teen cope*.

University of Florida Health. (2024). *Helping children cope with hospitalization*.

WakeMed Health & Hospitals. (2024). *Tips for hospitalized infants*.

WakeMed Health & Hospitals. (2024). *Tips for hospitalized preschoolers*.

WakeMed Health & Hospitals. (2024). *Tips for hospitalized school age children*.

WakeMed Health & Hospitals. (2024). *Tips for hospitalized adolescents*.

Williams, N.A., Brik, A.B., Petkus, J.M., & Clark, H. (2019). Importance of play for young children facing illness and hospitalization: Rationale, opportunities, and a case study illustration. *Early Child Development and Care*. https://doi/10.10/03004430.2019.1601088

Notes

Notes

Notes

Notes

Notes

Notes